Migraines: The Complete Guide

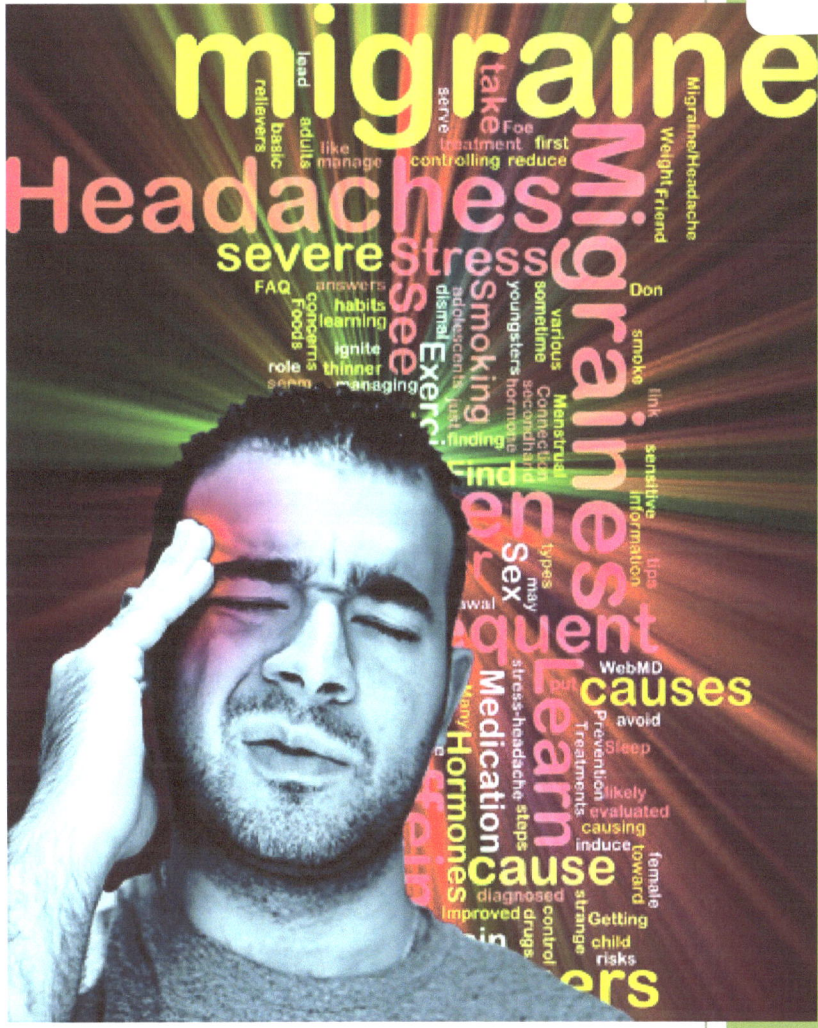

T. Godwin

TABLE OF CONTENTS:

Forward:

I have been a migraine sufferer for over 20 years now. I had my first migraine when I was 23 years old. I had a throbbing pain above my right eye, light hurt my eyes and I was throwing up. I thought I had a virus until I kept having the same thing over and over. I went to my doctor who gave me a neural exam. When she was complete, she told me they were migraines and gave me Midrin for them. No one else in my family has migraines and they just started happening out of left field. I didn't really know what they were or how they would affect the rest of my life. I wanted to write this complete guide on migraines so that others would be able to get an overall view of what migraines are, what to expect from them and ways to treat them. I thank you for purchasing this book and I hope it helps un-muddy the waters, so to speak.

Best regards,
T. Godwin
Author

Introduction:

More than 30 million Americans suffer from migraine headaches which can be classified as severe and often disabling headaches. A typical migraine headache will give a warning sign before its onset, such as tingling in your limbs, seeing blind spots or flashing lights. You will know when you are experiencing a migraine headache because they are accompanied by most, if not all of the following symptoms. Severe pain either on one side or both sides of the head, pulsing head pain, worsening head pain with any activity, nausea or vomiting, sensitivity to light and sound, and not being able to function regularly. While seeing flashing lights or blind spots are a common warning sign of a migraine, some sufferers experience these symptoms throughout the entire duration of their headache. This is classified as a classic migraine. Along with the above conditions, the person will also experience weakness and speech problems along with zigzagging lines in their eyes. If a migraine is left untreated, the pain can last from four to 72 hours, which can cause huge disturbances in a person's normal life.

Although doctors are not 100 percent sure what causes migraines to occur, there are some things that are known to trigger these headaches. Many women claim that their migraines worsen just before a period or during menopause and pregnancy. Certain foods can also trigger migraines, such as alcohol, cheese, chocolate, aspartame and caffeine. To avoid migraines as best you can, try keeping a diary of the foods you eat and record how they made you feel afterwards. After a couple of weeks doing this you should be able to see what foods are triggers for you, therefore telling you which foods to avoid. Other triggers can include stress, changes in the environment and certain medications.

To prevent migraines try avoiding trigger foods, as well as exercise regularly, cutting down on estrogen producing drugs if you are a woman, and quitting smoking and drinking alcohol. All of these things can help you avoid migraines, but if you do happen to get one, try over the counter pain medications or talk to you doctor about prescription drugs that are right for you.

Chapter 1: Migraine Stages

Migraines develop in four stages. Patients with migraines with aura, also known as classic migraines, are most likely to experience all four stages. Patients who have common migraines, migraines without aura, will have the same stages, but are not consciously aware of them. The interval between migraines is sometimes referred to as the fifth stage of a migraine.

Stage One – Prodrome
The prodromal phase usually begins one or two days prior to the actual migraine headache. Many migraine sufferers call this the "premonition" phase. Feelings during this phase are all over the map. Each migraine sufferer has their own personal prodrome profile. Some are giddy, happy, and full of energy, far more so than usual. Others feel a headache start with fatigue, weakness, and irritability. Anything can herald a migraine and each person has to learn their own prodrome signs if they want to learn to stave off the migraine.

Stage Two – Aura
This phase is skipped by most migraine sufferers, since most migraine sufferers suffer from common migraine, migraine without aura. For those who experience classic migraine with aura, auras can begin anywhere from five minutes to an hour before the headache begins. Auras are visual effects migraine sufferers often experience. Objects appear to have bright auras or haloes around them. Lightning flashes arc over the field of vision until sight is whited out just before the pain begins.

Stage Three - Headache
This phase lasts anywhere from four to seventy-two hours. Most common is a one-sided headache with a throbbing or pulsing characteristic. The headache is frequently accompanied by stomach upset, nausea, vomiting, and sensitivity to light, sound, smell, or some combination of the three.

Stage Four – Postdrome
Coming away from a migraine can be as unpleasant as building up to one. Postdrome is often characterized by tenderness of the head, neck, and stomach. Weakness and fatigue are also common in this phase.

Chapter 2: Migraine Criteria

The Classification Subcommittee of the International Headache Society (IHS) publishes and revises the "International Classification of Headache Disorders", now in its second edition. This book offers specific diagnostic criteria for diagnosing migraines and is currently used worldwide.

According to IHS, a common migraine headache, also known as a migraine without aura, is defined by the specific criteria found below.

Frequency
The patient must have at least five of these headaches.

Duration
The headache, excluding attendant symptoms or prodromes, must last a minimum of four hours, up to seventy-two hours. Headaches that last over seventy-two hours generally require immediate medical attention in order to rule out other, more dangerous conditions.

Pain Descriptors
In order to be classed as a migraine a headache must include at least two of four different qualities of pain:
1) The pain is one-sided; the headache is primarily on one side of the head.
2) The pain is not constant; it throbs, pounds, or pulsates.
3) The pain must be of moderate or severe intensity, to the point where the sufferer is inhibited in daily activity, potentially to the point of being temporarily disabled.
4) The pain is increased, sometimes only slightly, by routine physical activity like bending over, climbing stairs, or moving quickly.

Side Effects
Headache pain must be accompanied at least one of four common side effects:
1) Nausea
2) Vomiting
3) Photophobia – sensitivity to light
4) Phonophobia – sensitivity to sound

Secondary Exclusions
To rule out other conditions that may have caused the headache appropriate medical testing, such as a MRI, CAT scan, and/or a physician's exam must be conducted.

These criteria have helped simplify the diagnosis of migraine for many. However, because migraines are historically associated with extremely high levels of pain, people suffering from moderate migraine may not realize that is what they are experiencing.

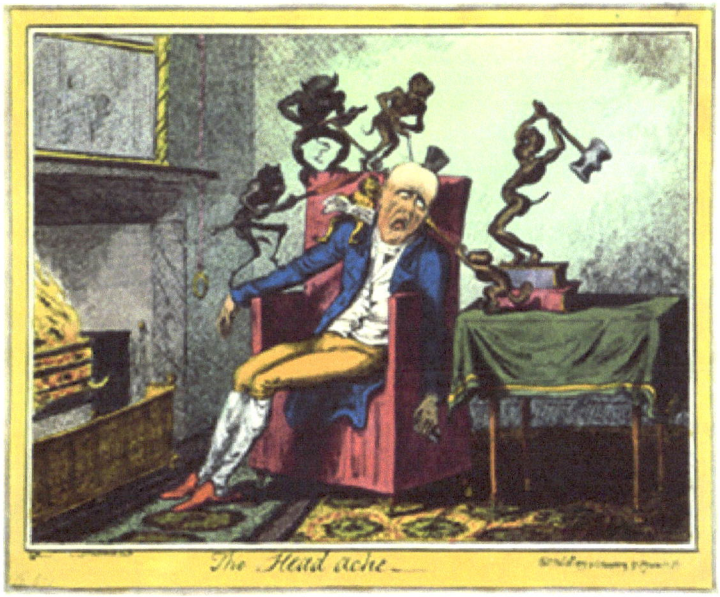

Chapter 3: Migraine Myths

There are a number of commonly held beliefs about migraines that make it hard for sufferers to get proper diagnosis and treatment.

1) Migraines are not real (all in the head, an overreaction to a normal headache, etc.).
Not true. Migraines are a biologic primary headache disorder. Even migraine pain is not confined to the head, though that is generally where it is worst.

2) Migraines have a known cause.
No, sadly not. There have been several interesting theories put forward in the last decade, but no single, definitive biological cause of migraines has been identified thus far.

3) All migraine sufferers have the same symptoms.
No, they don't. This is one of the things that makes migraines so hard to diagnose, particularly if a patient's doctor is only familiar with the most common symptoms.

4) A doctor can tell if it's a migraine or not.
Not always. The wide spectrum of symptoms that can accompany migraine can make it difficult to diagnose, more so if the patient is not forthcoming with their doctor about all their symptoms.

5) Migraines are curable.
No, they are not. Once properly diagosed many migraine sufferers still have to devote a lot of time and energy to managing their condition through medications, natural and homeopathic remedies, and diet and lifestyle changes. The various available coping methods work differently for each individual, so there is not even a single protocol of care.

6) Migraines are a woman's headache.
Women migraine sufferers do outnumber the men 3 to 1, but there is no evidence the condition is sex-linked in any way.

7) Only adults get migraines.
Migraines have been diagnosed in adolescents, children, and even infants.

8) Every headache a migraine sufferer has is a migraine
Not true. Migraine sufferers can have regular sinus, tension, or stress headaches just like anyone else.

Chapter 4: Are You In Or Out?

You have a migraine. You have a job. Now what do you do?

Deciding if you are able to go out when you have a migraine is a tough decision. If you're in pain and not feeling well, you're likely to not be thinking clearly. The ability to determine when you are okay to leave home when you have a migraine is a big part of learning to manage your condition. Here are a few things to take into consideration when deciding if you are in or out for the day.

How do you feel?

Yes, you have a migraine, but can you function? Only you know your personal headache pattern, is it likely to get better or worse from where it is now? What's your mood? Are you sufficiently enthused about the day to be willing to function while in pain?

What did you take?

Stop and think about your pain relief for a minute. Did you take an over-the-counter remedy, or something a little stronger? If it was a prescription medication, go read the label and see what it says about driving and operating heavy machinery. If you aren't supposed to do those things, it's probably a good idea to hang out at home. This is not a hard and fast rule since only you know how you react to a medicine, particularly one you are familiar with. If you don't think you"ll be impaired by your medications, great, but really think about it first.

Why?

Why are you going out? Basically, you have to decide how important it is that you go out. Work is important, but not if you have a job where potentially impaired function can be dangerous. Errands can always be run later. The class play? That might be worth it, if you can handle it.

Chapter 5: The High Price of Migraines

Migraines are expensive. Recent studies show that the chronic, debilitating headaches have a high cost not just for the sufferer, but for their family, and, surprisingly, their employer as well.

Migraine sufferers pay an enormous quality of life cost. Their wallets suffer as well. Health care costs for families with a migraine sufferer are, on average, seventy percent higher than those of families without a migraine sufferer. Migraine sufferers also pay for their pain in lost income. Sometime this is due to unpaid time away from work. Sadly, at other times it is because raises and promotions are not made available to them because they are deemed unreliable due to their condition.

The costs to employers are high, too. In the United States, it is estimated that migraines cost employers over twenty-four billion dollars each year. Half of that amount is indirect costs, things like absenteeism, short-term disability, and worker's compensation. It is estimated that these costs would be even higher if "presenteeism" were included. Presenteeism is the estimated cost of lost productivity that employees with migraines experience while on the job.

Of the estimated twelve point seven billion dollars migraines cost employers directly each year, the number one expense contributor is outpatient care. Outpatient care for migraines costs employers an estimated $6.2 billion annually. It is followed closely by prescription drug costs at $5.2 billion per year, and the remaining percentage is split between inpatient care and emergency costs.

This is not just a U.S. problem. In the United Kingdom, an estimated twenty-five million working or school days are lost annually due to migraines. Costs of absenteeism and lost productivity have gotten so high that employers are being asked to encourage migraine sufferer employees to seek treatment as a cost-saving measure.

Chapter 6: Home for Headaches

When a migraine strikes, many migraine sufferers head for home and settle in to wait out the excruciating headache. This may be the problem. While current genetic studies of rare migraines types show the condition to be about sixty percent inherited, the other forty is environmental. If someone already prone to migraines is exposed to an environmental trigger, fireworks, or at least a few prodromal symptoms, will ensue.

How can migraine sufferers make sure their homes aren't giving them headaches? Clear out known offenders, one at a time. Things to look out for:

* Common household allergens, things like mold, mildew, and dust and dust mites. Changing the air filter and switching to cotton sheets both help with these household horrors.

* Tobacco smoke. Whether it's a cigarette or a pipe, ask smokers to take it outside.

* Carbon monoxide. This odorless, colorless, and poisonous gas can come from poorly ventilated fireplaces, furnaces, gas appliances, or cars running in the garage. Installing carbon monoxide detectors near possible carbon monoxide sources and checking the batteries regularly may not only prevent migraines, it may save a life.

* Water-borne impurities. Eliminating potential chemical trouble from the faucet can be as simple as purchasing a small water filtering pitcher for drinking water. For extremely sensitive people a household filtration or softener system may be the answer.

* Pesticides. No one wants to share their home with insects and rodents, but the chemicals used to repel them may be inviting in migraines. Temporarily eliminating pesticide use or switching to organic pest control may help.

* Pet dander. Migraine sufferers who are allergic to their pet may want to consider allergy treatment to help them live with the problem.

* Cleaning solutions. The number and variety of harsh chemicals found in cleansers is boggling. Switching to all-natural cleansers may clean up migraines.

Chapter 7: Migraine Prodromes

A migraine prodrome is a premonition or advance warning that a migraine is coming on. Prodromes can occur anywhere from a few minutes before the onset of a headache to days prior. While no one knows the specific cause of migraine prodromes, the prevailing theory is that they are part of neurochemical change in the brain that occurs before an attack. Approximately 60% of all migraine sufferers (people who have chronic migraines) experience some type of prodrome.

Migraine Auras

Migraine auras are a specific type of visual prodrome in which people see things that are not there, like flashes of light or haloes around object. This type of prodrome is rare and experienced by less than 25% of all migraine sufferers.

Emotional Changes

Many migraine sufferers describe mood alterations preceding an attack. Some people are euphoric, others fall into a profound despondence, and still others experience uncharacteristic irritability or impatience.

Metabolic Changes

Some migraine sufferers describe their prodrome experience as an enormous spike in energy levels during the day preceding the headache itself. Others say that they know a migraine is coming because they get fatigued or listless or find themselves constantly yawning prior to onset.

Appetite Changes

Some migraine sufferers lose their appetite before a headache. Some sufferers find themselves ravenous the day or night before an attack. Still others have noticed that specific cravings tend to precede their migraine.

Sleep Changes

Insomnia is a frequent prodrome symptom for many migraine sufferers, as is difficulty falling asleep. Others experience lassitude and difficulty waking prior to a migraine.

Migraines are often difficult to diagnose and treat because no two migraine patients experience the same prodromes, if they experience one at all. Many migraine sufferers experience all of the prodrome symptoms at different times before a single headache, or different ones prior to different attacks.

Chapter 8: Migraine Auras

A migraine aura is a specific type of prodrome (or premonition) that heralds a migraine. It is a symptom or series of symptoms that let migraine sufferers, people who suffer from chronic migraines, know in advance that a migraine headache is about to make itself felt.

Aura effects develop over about five minutes and generally occur from twenty minutes to an hour prior to the start of a headache. They are a symptom of what used to be called "classic migraine". Recently, medical practitioners have moved to a more scientifically accurate term, migraine-with-aura. Only about 15-20% of migraine sufferers consistently experience any kind of aura before a headache begins.

Aura Effects

Most migraine auras are visual. These auras are called positive visual phenomena because, rather than their vision fading or going dark, people who experience them see things. Examples include:

-Auras or Haloes: a nimbus of light or haze surrounding objects, particularly light sources

-Flashing or Floating Lights: colored or white (rarely dark) spots that appear to move

-Lightning Bolts: a jagged or zigzag line that sparkles and/or arcs over the field of vision; with the frequency or severity increasing over time until the person can no longer see (a whiteout); This effect usually stops with the onset of headache pain.

-Photophobia: an extreme sensitivity to light; this effect frequently lasts the duration of the headache

Most auras last less than an hour. Migraine sufferers who experience auras that last more than an hour are said to suffer from migraines with prolonged aura. In some cases a migraine sufferer may experience aura effects without a headache developing, but it is still considered to be a symptom of chronic migraines. At various times the same person may experience all three variations, migraine with aura, migraine with prolonged aura, or typical aura without headache.

Chapter 9: Abdominal Migraines

Anyone who has ever had a migraine will say they do not just happen in the head. The headache is usually the worst and most painful part of a migraine, but there's more. Most migraine sufferers (people who suffer from migraines) will talk about photosensitivity (sensitivity to light), phonosensitivity (sensitivity to sound), scent sensitivity, gastric pain, cramping, and vomiting.

Sometimes the abdominal symptoms show up without the other typical migraine symptoms. When they do, a patient is said to be experiencing an abdominal migraine. An abdominal migraine is pain, usually varying from mild to medium, in the abdomen. The pain is either along the midline or unspecified and is frequently accompanied by abdominal tenderness, cramp-like spasms, bloating, vomiting, and loss of appetite.

Since abdomen pain can be caused by a wide variety of conditions other causes need to be ruled out before a diagnosis can be made. In a classic abdominal migraine, no gastric cause for the pain can be identified. Migraine sufferers need to let their doctors know about their migraines when they experience unspecified abdominal pain so that the doctor knows abdominal migraine may be a possibility.

Abdominal migraines are most common in children. Children who experience abdominal migraines frequently grow up to be migraine sufferers. While abdominal migraine is not unheard of in adults, it is rare. Like most other types of migraine, it is also more common in females than in males.

While the exact cause of abdominal migraines is unknown, it is highly likely to be related to serotonin deficiency. Serotonin deficiency has been linked in several studies to migraines, and 90% of the body's serotonin is produced in the gastric system. Serotonin deficiency causes cascading waves of nerve reaction in the brain when triggering a migraine and a similar process may be in effect in the abdomen.

Chapter 10: Hemiplegic Migraine

There are a number of different types of migraine headaches, including both the classic and common migraine. One particularly rare type of migraine is the hemiplegic migraine.

Hemiplegic migraines are migraine headaches with very particular symptoms.

They include:
* A sudden attack unilateral (one-sided) weakness and/or paralysis, typically during the aura phase of migraine.
* The weakness frequently involves a migraine sufferers face, arm, and leg.
* When the right side of the body is the affected side, the migraine sufferer may be speech impaired.
* A mild head trauma can trigger a hemiplegic migraine.
* A migraine headache follows the paralysis.
* The paralysis lasts from an hour to days, but usually clears up within 24 hours.
* Dizziness, vertigo, double vision, and difficulty in walking or balancing may all be part of a hemiplegic migraine.

Hemiplegic migraines are predominantly genetic and sufferers usually have at least one first or second-degree relative (parent, sibling, aunt, uncle, first cousin) who also suffers from hemiplegic migraines. Since many hemiplegic migraines are brought on by minor head trauma, people with a propensity for this type of migraine are encouraged to avoid contact sports. In families where the condition is common, onset frequently occurs in childhood, so the no-contact rule is particularly important for children in hemiplegic prone families. Several genetic markers have been identified for hemiplegic migraine specifically. It is not a condition that screening is normally offered for, but screening is available for it upon request. This type of migraine is particularly disturbing because its symptoms so closely resemble a stroke. Fortunately, the stroke-like effects usually reverse completely within 24 hours. They are also problematic because hemiplegic migraines do not respond to most migraine medications and often have to be treated more like epilepsy with more dangerous medications than regular migraine sufferers take.

Chapter 11: Transformed Migraine

Migraine headaches bring some of the most excruciating pain a person will ever know. Many migraine sufferers say the only good thing about a migraine is the relief they feel when the headache is over. Knowing that a good feeling is waiting on the other side is the only thing that helps some get through the pain.

People who live with transformed migraine (TM) do not have anything to look forward to. Transformed migraine is the name of a condition some migraine sufferers develop after years of migraine episodes. Most people develop transformed migraines in their 20s or 30s.

Migraine sufferers report less severe headaches suddenly, but they come more often until they turn into chronic daily headaches (CDH). The daily headache is less intense than a migraine episode, but still painful, and most transformed migraine patients still have occasional full-blown migraine episodes.

Not all migraine sufferers will develop transformed migraines. In fact, most won't. Those who do are predominantly women and approximately 90% of them previously had migraine with aura (classic migraine). Migraine with aura is relatively rare, affecting less than 20% of all migraine sufferers.

The exact cause of transformed migraines is, like all migraine types, unknown. Many transformed migraine sufferers are heavy users of pain-relievers, both over the counter items like acetaminophen and naproxen and prescription medications like Vicodin or Darvon. Some even take them daily, whether they have a migraine or not, thinking they may help prophylactically.

TM patients of this type are particularly hard to treat because of a developed tolerance for pain medication. The first step in treating these patients is to wean them from their daily medications. Sometimes this step alone will stop the chronic lesser headaches. Once weaned, like non-medication dependent TM patients, their migraines are manageable with a regular treatment regimen just like any other migraine sufferer.

Chapter 12: Basilar Migraines

Migraines can be more than just a pain in the head. Basilar migraines, once known as basilar artery migraines or BAMs, are an extraordinarily rare but potentially life-threatening variant of the classic migraine with aura.

Basilar migraine symptoms are caused by constriction of the basilar artery, which supplies blood to the brain stem. BAMs were originally thought to affect only young women and adolescent girls, but research shows that while they are primarily a problem for these groups they can occur in people of all ages and genders.

During the aura phase, basilar migraine symptoms may include loss of balance, double vision or partial vision loss, lack of coordination, numbness on one or both sides of the body, weakness, dizziness or confusion and severe vomiting. The symptoms typically last an hour or less and disappear when the headache begins. Some basilar migraine sufferers pass out or lose consciousness during the aura phase as well. In extremely rare cases, they may even slip into a coma that can last hours or days.

The danger of basilar migraines is that they can lead to a transient ischemic attack (TIA) or stroke. A transient ischemic attack is essentially a miniature stroke resulting from a temporary interruption of the flow of blood to the brain. Unlike strokes, TIAs have not been shown to cause permanent damage to the brain and most neurological problems that arise from them, like slurred speech or weakness on one side, clear up within twenty-four hours of the attack.

The basilar artery is located at the back of head. The headache associated with basilar migraines is usually a severe throbbing ache on both sides of the back of the head, as opposed to the unilateral temple throbbing more commonly associated with migraines.

Chapter 13: Pediatric Migraines

Children get migraines too, it's not a condition confined to adulthood. Studies have even indicated that infants may get migraines, but this is hard to verify.

Current estimates indicate that up to 10% of children between 5-15 years old suffer from migraines, increasing to 28% in the 15-19 age range. Migraine headaches have a real impact on quality of life for children. The high percentage of children that experience migraines makes them a top childhood health problems.

Diagnosing pediatric migraine is similar to diagnosing adult migraines with a few notable exceptions. The International Headache Society's criteria states that the headache must last 4 to 72 hours. Children's migraines are generally shorter and this fact needs to be taken into account when attempting to diagnose them. Adult migraines are frequently one-sided, but children's frequently involve pain on both sides of the head. These headaches should not be dismissed just because they are not one-sided.

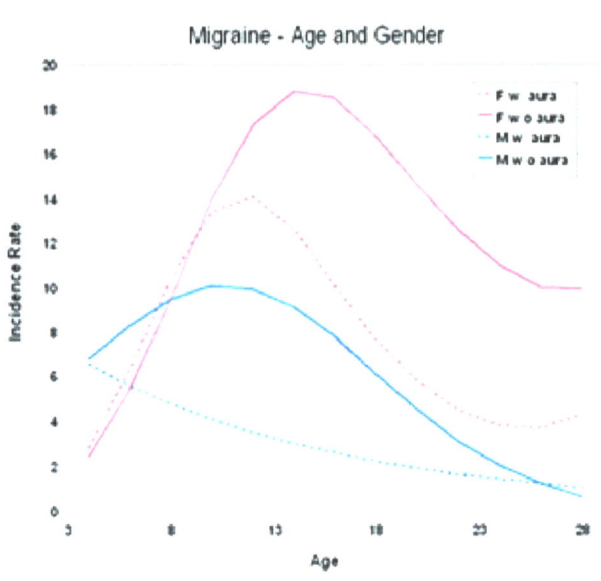

For most child migraine sufferers (people suffering from migrainous headaches) the headaches begin between 5 and 11 years of age. Prior to puberty, the number of male and female children with migraines is roughly equal. After puberty, girls are considerably more likely than boys are to have migraines, most likely due to the same hormonal issues that make the number of adult women migraine sufferers three times that of the men.

Many child migraine sufferers are fortunate enough to have their condition disappear during puberty or upon reaching adulthood. However, people who have migraines as children are much more likely to become adult migraine sufferers than those who did not have them as a child.

Adult migraine sufferers should watch for migraine symptoms in their children, particular if the other parent also experiences migraines. A child with two migraine sufferer parents has a 70% chance of becoming a migraine sufferer.

Chapter 14: Non-drug Treatment for Pediatric Migraine

The last thing most parents want to do is give their child a drug. Yet, when that child is a migraine sufferer (a person with chronic migraine headaches), as are a reported 10-28% of children under the age of 19, many feel they have no choice.

This is simply not true. In fact, most pediatric neurology specialists will recommend alternative treatments before medication for safety reasons. A number of non-drug therapies are available for pediatric migraine sufferers. As with any complementary or alternative medicine (CAM) treatment, the patient's physician must be a part of the team making the decisions and overseeing care.

One of the most common non-drug treatment options is temperature therapy. The application of a warm or cool compress eases pain for many. Apply the hot or cold pack to the area of greatest pain, taking care to insulate it so no damage to the child's skin occurs.

Sleep frequently eases the suffering of adult migraine sufferers. The duration of children's migraines is usually shorter than that of an adult. A nap taken in a dark, quiet, area can eliminate some migraines altogether.

Scheduling can be a factor in reducing the frequency of pediatric migraines. Unlike adults, who experience stress in an acute, episodic manner, children usually experience a constant stress level, particularly during the school year. Establishing a regular routine, including time to relax and an age-appropriate sleep schedule, helps many young migraine sufferers.

Relaxation training, including instruction in self-hypnosis and guided imagery, is becoming the treatment of choice for recurrent pediatric migraines. Studies show that over half of the pediatric patients who learn these relaxation techniques experience less frequent migraines, but with no reduction in pain intensity when they do have one.

There are many options for pediatric migraine therapy, do not be afraid to ask the doctor about drug alternatives.

Chapter 15: Common Migraine Food Triggers

No one knows for sure what causes migraine headaches. The most likely to answer to-date is that a serious of small irritations or reactions pile up until, finally, a migraine headache is triggered. Migraine triggers are different for each individual, but many migraine sufferers claim that a particular food or combination of foods will push them over the edge into a headache.

Keep in mind that most science disagrees with migraine sufferers when it comes to food triggers. There are no conclusive studies indicating a link between certain foods and migraine headaches, so all information is anecdotal. The thing is there is a lot, tons in fact, of anecdotal evidence for the link.

While a migraine trigger food can be, quite literally, anything, some foods come up on the trigger list for enough people to merit discussion.

Cheese
Cheese is a major trigger for many migraine sufferers. Particularly likely to cause an attack are hard or aged cheeses. Soft cheeses like cream cheese and new cheeses seem to be fine and unlikely to cause problems.

Processed Meats
Nitrates are believed by many to be a major migraine trigger. For most people, the most common source of nitrates is processed meat, items like hot dogs, sausage, bacon, processed lunchmeats, etc.

Condiments
Salad dressings are a trigger for many. The reason is not known, but is probably tied to a combination of other triggers all coming together in one place.

Spices and Additives
Any spice can be a trigger. Spices as triggers may be tied, at least partially, to scent sensitivity, since many spices have a pungent odor. Seasonings that seem to give migraine sufferers the most trouble include monosodium glutamate (MSG), common in Asian foods, artificial sweeteners, food dyes, and vinegar.

Migraine sufferers who suspect a food trigger should consider trying an elimination diet to pinpoint the trigger food(s).

Chapter 16: Migraines and Rebound Headaches

A rebound headache, also known as a medication overuse headache, is one of the most unpleasant side effects of migraines for many sufferers. These headaches are often blindingly painful, and are sometimes migraines in their own right.

How do people get rebound headaches? Put simply, they try just a little too hard to find relief from their migraine pain. The migraine sufferer is in pain and takes medication. They are still in pain later and take a little more. That does not help, so they try more medicine to relieve their suffering.

A rebound headache is when a migraine (or other severe headache) spins off into another headache as a result of medication overuse. A rebound headache is basically the original headache, which is only temporarily masked by all the drugs. When the body is finally clear of all the medications, the headache pain returns or rebounds.

Sometimes the rebound is a migraine or a continuation of the previous migraine. Others it is a blindingly painful new headache in its own right. The new headache is excruciatingly painful but without the additional symptoms, like nausea and photosensitivity, that often accompany migraines.

The overuse of any over-the-counter or prescription pain reliever can cause a rebound headache, but the two most frequent culprits are aspirin and acetaminophen. Other drugs often involved in the rebound cycle include caffeine, opiates, prescription combination medications like Midrin, codeine, ergotamine titrate, and drugs that contain barbiturates.

While all really painful, chronic headaches should be discussed with a doctor, there are a number of indicators that someone is probably suffering from medication overuse headaches. These include:

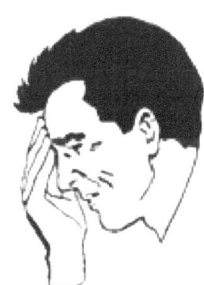

* daily or every other day headaches
* medications no longer provide the relief they used to
* prophylactic medication use

With the help of their doctor, rebound headache patients can break the cycle.

Chapter 17: Migraines and PMS

No one knows exactly what causes migraine headaches, or even what happens in the body and brain when someone has one. One thing that is known, however, is that three times as many women as men have migraines. Many female migraine sufferers will also confess that their headaches are likely to coincide with the period just before their menstrual period.

A whopping sixty percent of women migraine sufferers have migraines during their period and during the rest of the month. Fourteen percent only have a migraine headache during their period. Look at the numbers; seventy-four percent of all women migraine sufferers associate their period with their headaches, and while medical science does not deny the connection, the reason for it is still unknown.

In addition, many women who become migraine sufferers later in life say that their pre-menstrual syndrome (PMS) symptoms became much more acute since the headaches began. A study published in the January 2006 issue of Headache confirmed the apocryphal evidence. Women participating reported that bloating, weight gain, breast tenderness, mood swings, back pain, and abdominal cramps all became more severe during a migraine.

The women in the study were given a medication to induce a temporary artificial menopause by halting the action of the ovaries. Even with the hormonal ups and downs of regular periods eliminated, they still reported worsened PMS symptoms during a migraine attack.

The fourteen percent of women who only have migraines during their period are said to have "menstrual migraines". There is hope, though. For some lucky women, taking a brief course of NSAIDs (non-steroidal anti-inflammatory medicines, like ibuprofen) for several days prior to their period as well as the first few days of it can stave off a menstrual migraine. Women who want to try this type of prophylactic treatment should discuss the option with their doctor.

Chapter 18: Migraines and Obesity

Are you more likely to have migraines if you are obese?

The simple answer, for adults, is no.

The more complicated answer is sort-of. Obesity does not cause migraines in adults—the jury is still out on how obesity affects pediatric migraine

That's the good news. The bad news is that migraine and obesity can have a devastating effect on each other.

While obesity does not cause migraines, migraines, especially for people with migraines plus chronic daily headaches, can lead to obesity. People with migraines are likely to spend more time being sedentary, forced to inaction by the pain in their head. Additionally, many medications given to migraine sufferers cause weight gain directly, others cause it indirectly by increasing appetite.

Weight gain leads to depression in many people, which leads to more unhealthy behaviors (compulsiveness, hopelessness, increased inactivity, etc.) Inaction, weight gain, and increased appetite—a road that begins in migraine may well end in obesity.

Recent studies have divided migraine sufferers into different categories by their body mass index (BMI). The higher the body mass index, the more overweight the patient. The majority of the study participants were women, and median age was approximately 38 years.

Obese migraine sufferers, those with a BMI of 30 or higher, are far more likely to have extra problems with their migraines than people with a lower BMI are. Patients with higher body mass indexes reported more frequent headaches that lasted longer and were more severe than those experienced by lower BMI patients were.

There have been several studies on weight and headache prevalence, especially migraines, in children and teens. The initial results are a little frightening since almost all of them saw a correlation between a high BMI and incidence of migraines and other types of severe headaches (tension headaches, cluster headaches). All agreed, however, that more research is needed.

Chapter 19: Migraines and Caffeine

Migraine sufferers have a love-hate relationship with caffeine. For many, the vasoconstrictor helps alleviate their migraine pain. For an equal number, the chemical is a migraine headache trigger. The relationship between caffeine and migraines is anything but straightforward.

For caffeine addicts who discover that their daily cup is a migraine trigger the problem of caffeine is particularly thorny. People who regularly consume large quantities of caffeine often experience withdrawal headaches if they do not get their regular java jolt. If they are predisposed to migraines, the headache they get if they cut out the caffeine is going to be a doozy. Many people think caffeine withdrawal alone can bring on a migraine. Regular caffeine-aholics are advised to lower their caffeine intake slowly so they do not send their body into withdrawal.

Many migraine pain relievers include caffeine. The vasoconstrictive action of caffeine helps relieve migraine pain for some people. One current theory of what exactly goes on in the head during migraine proposes that arteries in the temple get inflamed during an attack and vasoconstriction would reduce the inflammation. Another possible reason to include caffeine in a migraine medication is because it acts as a supplement to the main analgesic. Studies have shown that many analgesics function more efficiently and pack a greater punch when paired with caffeine, though no one is sure exactly why.

Caffeine shows up in many unexpected places, so migraine sufferers who are sensitive to it (not all are) need to be vigilant label readers. Everyone knows about beverages, things like coffee and colas. Caffeine is also found in many clear or fruit-flavored sodas. Caffeine can be found in chocolate; the darker the chocolate the more caffeine it contains. Caffeine is in many over-the-counter analgesics, and not always clearly labeled. Migraine sufferers should be especially wary of caffeine in over-the-counter migraine formulas of regular medications.

Chapter 20: Migraines and Insomnia

A bout of insomnia will often bring on a migraine in someone prone to them. Having a migraine will often lead to insomnia. It sounds like a vicious cycle, and, for some migraine sufferers, it can be.

Insomnia is characterized by the inability to fall asleep, stay asleep, or fall back to sleep if awakened unexpectedly. Head and abdominal pain from a migraine may exacerbate the inability to sleep in people already inclined to sleep disorders. A 2005 study published in Headache, the journal of the American Headache Society, discusses the links between poor sleep and migraines. Most of the study participants reported some form of sleep trouble and over 50% attributed migraine onset to sleep disturbances at least some of the time. Almost 40% of participants admitted to sleeping six or less hours a night. These "short sleepers" experienced more frequent and severe migraines than other migraine sufferers. Short sleepers were also more likely to wake up with daily headaches, a condition known as transformed migraines. Over 85% of the study participants said they chose to sleep or rest because of headache pain and 75% said the pain forced them to sleep. Insomnia and migraines have something in common. Serotonin deficiency is linked to a number of disorders, including migraines and insomnia. Serotonin is a neurotransmitter thought to be an important part of the body's regulation of sleep, mood, appetite, vomiting, and body temperature. It is manufactured in the gastrointestinal tract, where 90% of it is produced, and the central nervous system, and then stored in the blood.

Insufficient serotonin levels are also associated with several gastric disorders. This may explain why so many migraine sufferers experience stomach problems prior to or during a headache. Lack of serotonin is also likely to be a major component in the phenomenon known as abdominal migraines.

Chapter 21: Migraines and Depression

Being in pain so fierce that the only recourse is to hide in a dark, quiet room until it is over several times a year would make anyone sad. Migraine sufferers, though, are five times more likely to develop clinical depression than people who do not have these debilitating headaches. Conversely, people who are depressed are three times likelier than happy people to become migraine sufferers.

Many scientists view the intertwining of migraine and depression as a chicken or egg situation. They are patently comorbid, but does one cause the other? If so, which one starts the process, the migraine or the depression? The answer is not that simple. Migraines, depression, and, unsurprisingly, insomnia, a state associated with both conditions have something in common. All three are associated with neurotransmitter deficiencies in the brain.

Doctors believe that while they are related, depression and migraine headaches have distinct causes with a similar neurobiology. For years, doctors blamed depression in migraine sufferers on their resultant loss of quality of life due to headaches. Now it looks as though the link is a biologic shared mechanism rather than psychology.

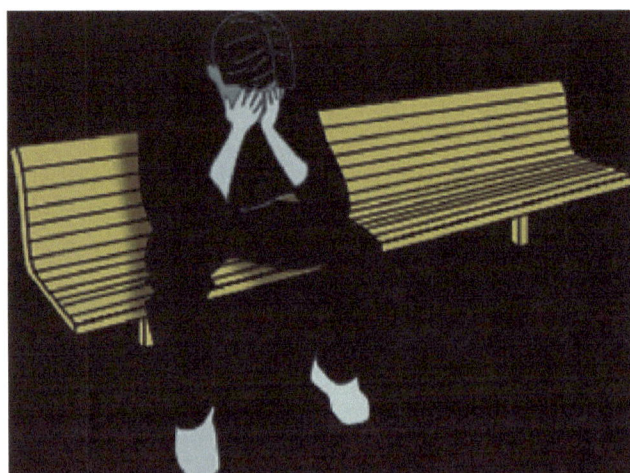

One danger for clinically depressed migraine sufferers is possible drug interaction between their depression medication and their migraine drugs. In July 2006 the FDA recognized one such danger, that of mixing triptans for migraines with SSRIs (selective serotonin reuptake inhibitors) or SNRIs (serotonin and norepinephrine reuptake inhibitors), used to treat depression and mood disorders. Combining the drugs can lead to a condition called serotonin syndrome.

Serotonin syndrome occurs when there is too much serotonin in the body. Symptoms include hallucinations, increased heart rate and body temperature, fast changes in blood pressure, and gastrointestinal upset. Sometimes a patient has no choice but to take these medications together, but they need to weigh their options with their doctor and be monitored closely for serotonin syndrome.

Chapter 22: Aging and Migraines

Aging is a fact of life. Getting older means increasing frailty and susceptibility to illness, but it can also be a boon to migraine sufferers (people who experience migraine headaches). Only 2-10% of the elderly population experiences migraines (as opposed to up to 28% of adults under 65), and elderly women are still more likely to have them than their male counterparts.

Migraines can happen at any age, but they peak around age 40. The frequency of migraine attacks after 40 decreases for most people. Many migraine sufferers who have suffered with this condition for years experience a reduction in the frequency and severity of attacks after age 55.

About two thirds of migraine sufferers stop having attacks altogether by age 65. Patients over 65 who still have migraines report drastically decreased severity, duration, and frequency in their attacks. They are also less likely to experience the gastrointestinal upset that accompanies migraine in younger people.

The downside to all this good news is that adults over 65 who suffer from migraines are more likely than younger patients to experience disability because of their affliction. Many physicians are uncomfortable with treating senior citizens for migraines because therapeutic methods used on younger people are often not tested for safety in an older patient.

Additional conditions and the medications used to treat them complicate the problem. Seniors are more likely to be on one or more prescription drugs and each new medication increases the risk of adverse drug reactions. This possibility makes some doctors reluctant to offer senior migraine sufferers pharmaceutical assistance.

The onset of migraines after age 50 is very rare and should be investigated with a doctor to rule out the possibility of secondary causes. Late onset does not rule out migraine (only one third of senior headaches are due to secondary conditions) but it makes it less likely.

Chapter 23: Smoking and Migraines

Is there a connection between smoking and migraines?

The correct answer is "maybe" to "probably". There is currently no study data specifically addressing this issue. Studies of smoking and chronic headaches in general (not all chronic headaches are migraines) are available, but their application to migraines is limited.

A study of smoking and patients with chronic cluster headaches yielded some telling results. Smoking patients who decreased their smoking by less than a half of a pack daily reduced their headache frequency by an amazing 50%. This study just asked patients to cut down n their smoking, not to eliminate it. Imagine the results that might have been achieved if the smokers quit entirely!

In another study, 53% of migraine patients who eliminated smoking in conjunction with the elimination of personally identified food triggers experienced a complete cessation of migraines. By contrast, only 13% of non-smoking patients who eliminated their food triggers became migraine-free.

Many migraine sufferers (people who suffer from migraine headaches) are sensitive to strong smells, like perfume, food odors, and, yes, tobacco smoke. Others are specifically sensitive only to the scent of tobacco smoke. Still others are allergic to cigarette, cigar, and pipe smoke.

All of these people report having smoking or secondhand smoke trigger a migraine. Sometimes the smoke is the only trigger, sometimes it is part of a combination of triggers. Experts and sufferers agree there must be a link between smoking and migraines, somewhere, waiting to be uncovered. Many of the commonly known effects of smoking are particularly detrimental to those prone to headaches and head pain. These side effects include elevated blood pressure, inflammation or irritation of the sinus cavities and nasal passages, and higher risk of stroke. Health officials all agree on one thing, smoking is contraindicated for everyone in every situation and migraine sufferers are no exception.

Chapter 24: Running Into Migraines

Exercise is good for you. Being fit will help your whole body feel better, including your migraines, right? So why did your headache specialist just tell you to drop out of this weekend's 10K if you want to be able to go to work on Monday?

A regular exercise program is a great migraine deterrent, but it needs to be the right kind of exercise. Many workout types put a real strain on the cardiovascular system and scientists have linked migraines to vascular problems in the temporal artery, among other potential causes.

Migraine sufferers who want to sweat need to warm up, slowly, for about fifteen minutes prior to any strenuous exertion, whether it is exercise or home repair. Skipping this warm up is nearly a guarantee that a migraine will be interrupting your plans later in the day.

While any exertion can be good or bad and each migraine sufferer is different, there are a few types of exercise that are notorious for bringing down the head.

* Aerobics: high-intensity aerobics classes are a trigger for many women, especially when the cardio-pounding workout is paired with loud music.
* Biking: Whether it is competitive cycling or spinning class at the club, this is a major trigger for many.
* Running: Any kind of running that involves hard-core exertion, especially endurance events like marathons and triathlons.

You may be able to keep doing these things, especially if you really enjoy them, but you need to think about toning down the endurance aspect. Cycling should be for pleasure and exercise but not competitive. Replace high impact aerobics classes with dance, yoga, or free weight aerobics. Reduce the distance you run and see if it helps with the migraines. There is no reason a migraine sufferer cannot be fit, just be careful to not get a migraine.

Chapter 25: Acupuncture for Migraines

Acupuncture is one of the oldest medical techniques in the world, practiced in China for over 2,000 years. It is a FDA-approved treatment modality for a number of illnesses, especially pain management and chronic pain, and is particularly effective in treating migraines.

Acupuncture is a Traditional Chinese Medicine treatment that involves stimulating some of the over 800 vital energy points in the human body with fine, hair-thin needles to release chi and encourage the body to heal itself. The vital energy points are on the meridians that run through the body from head to toe.

Chi (pronounced chee), or life energy, flows through these meridians and energy points. The obstruction of the flow of chi leads to illness and is considered the source of many bodily aches and pains. The flow of chi along the meridians can be obstructed by illness, poor diet, the weather, and other outside factors.

Most acupuncture practitioners work with patients to form a treatment plan that addresses both the blockages themselves and the things that cause them. The treatment plans, like those of Western Medicine, often include diet and lifestyle changes to enhance the patient's well-being.

Migraine sufferers need to tell their acupuncturist exactly where they hurt when seeing one for pain mitigation. The location of pain is important due to the large number of acupuncture points in the head, face, and neck. Where to apply pressure depends on where the migraine pain is most acute.

Migraine sufferers can find long-term relief from their migraines by working with an acupuncturist who specializes in headaches. These specialists do an individualized assessment of the patient to create a long-term treatment plan. Many people who undergo an acupuncture program like this experience relief from migraines for years afterward. For some the headaches stop completely.

Chapter 26: Acupressure and Migraines

Acupressure is a completely non-invasive treatment option that has a high success rate among migraine sufferers. It has a proven track record as a successful pain abatement technique. Acupressure is also efficacious in reducing both the frequency and intensity of migraine attacks.

In Traditional Chinese Medicine, there are over 800 vital energy points in the human body. These points lie along meridians that run throughout a person's body. Chi, or life energy, flows along the meridians and through the energy points in healthy people. Chi that is blocked or overabundant near particular energy points causes illness and pain. Acupressure massage applies pressure to these energy points in order to release chi and stimulate the body's own healing mechanisms. The energy points are massaged with the fingers, thumb, or occasional blunt object with medium pressure in a circular pattern. The simplest acupressure a migraine sufferer can learn is an all-over head massage. This technique just requires the practitioner to massage the scalp as though they were washing their hair. Sit with the elbows resting on a table to prevent arm strain and the head resting lightly in the hands to perform head and neck acupressure.

Moderate pressure applied to the GB20 points offers the best relief for migraine pain. They are on either side of the neck, approximately one inch to each side of the spinal column just below where the skull and neck muscles connect. GB20 also goes by the more romantic-sounding Chinese name "The Gates of Consciousness".

Migraine sufferers seeking to relieve their headache and neck pain should practice deep breathing while using the thumbs of both hands to press firmly on the GB20 points for one to two minutes. If this is painful at first, home practitioners can start out by pressing and releasing the points in five to fifteen second intervals.

Chapter 27: Aromatherapy and Migraines

Most physicians agree that aromatherapy makes an excellent complementary therapy for migraine sufferers. Aromatherapy has not been shown to eliminate migraine headaches, but when used to complement traditional therapy and medication it can reduce the frequency and severity of attacks.

Aromatherapy is a natural healing methodology that uses plant-derived essential oils to achieve a desired therapeutic effect. It is not known precisely how aromatherapy works, whether it is the scent or a chemical action of the essential oil itself that provides relief. Because of this unknown factor some doctor's worry about potential essential oil interactions with standard drugs used in treating migraines.

When trying aromatherapy to relieve migraines, keep in mind a few safety precautions.

* Always talk to a doctor before trying anything new.
* Speak to an experienced aromatherapist, if possible.
* When combining aromatherapy with other medications, watch for adverse reactions and report them to a doctor immediately.
* Buy real plant-derived essential oils designed for aromatherapy. Good ones will be sold in dark containers and stored away from direct sunlight.
* Use a carrier oil or aromatherapy diffuser. Essential oils can be powerful irritants and should not be applied directly to the skin.

Essential oils can be used in a number of ways. They can be used in an aromatherapy diffuser and inhaled two or three times daily. Oils can added to a large bowl of hot water and the aroma inhaled with eyes closed. While essential oils can also be added to carrier bath, face, or massage oils and applied to the body or bath, this should only be done after consulting with a knowledgeable aromatherapist to make sure the oils used are safe for this purpose.

Some of the essential oils commonly recommended for migraine aromatherapy are lavender, peppermint, rosemary, eucalyptus, sandalwood, clary sage, ginger, ylang-ylang, basil, marjoram, and chamomile.

Chapter 28: Neurostimulator Implants and Migraines

One out of every eight people suffers from migraine headaches. There is currently no treatment available to eliminate the condition; doctors merely help patients manage the symptoms. A new treatment is being tested that may offer more pain relief than any other method to date for migraine sufferers.

In September 2006, reports began surfacing about a surgical procedure that may help migraine sufferers. Dr. Sandeep Amin, an anesthesiologist at Rush University Medical Centre in Chicago, Illinois, is pioneering a radical new treatment.

Dr. Amin is studying the potential of a treatment he calls "occipital nerve stimulation". The treatment calls for the implantation of a small neurostimulator in the neck. This device sends electrical impulses to nerves under the skin at the base of the head at the back of the neck.

The device being used Dr. Amin's nationwide double-blind study is the Boston Scientific Precision neurostimulator. The Precision neurostimulator is the smallest rechargeable, implantable neurostimulator on the market (as of 2006) and is already FDA-approved for spinal stimulation for chronic pain treatment.

If the study is successful, it offers new hope to migraine sufferers, particularly those who have found their pain resistant to currently available treatment modalities.

Dr. Amin's study is not the first. In 2004, Medtronic, Inc., a medical technology company, conducted a study of occipital nerve stimulation for migraines using one of their own devices. The study was initiated after a Dallas doctor successfully used the experimental treatment to relieve pain for a migraine sufferer. A review of the company's website, www.medtronic.com, showed no information on the study, making it likely that, for whatever reason, the 2004 study was unsuccessful.

Dr. Amin states that his treatment is not for everyone, and, if it is successful, recommends it only for patients who have been unable to achieve pain relief through medication or other, more common, treatment methods.

Chapter 29: Yoga for Migraines

Stretching, breathing, bending—none of these activities sound good to a migraine sufferer in the throes of a headache, but they should.

Yoga is a physical and psychological discipline originating in India. Most modern yoga practiced in the West is hatha yoga, which is primarily concerned with asanas (postures), pranayama (breathing exercises), and meditation. Yoga is an excellent way to relieve stress, a common migraine trigger, and tone the body. Being active in a regular, low impact fitness program helps many migraine sufferers reduce the frequency and severity of their headaches. This makes yoga a good fit for migraine sufferers who want both less headaches and less pain medication in their lives.

As with any fitness plan, migraine sufferers need to consult their doctor before beginning a yoga regimen. Home fitness videos and books are great resources for beginners, but should not be the only resources a migraine sufferer uses when starting yoga. Many poses may actually increase the likelihood of headaches. Migraine sufferers who are seriously planning to take up yoga as a complement to their migraine treatment plan should make an appointment with a skilled yoga instructor to discuss their condition and what poses are appropriate. If they have a book, they should bring it to the appointment to review with the instructor.

For migraine sufferers who are thinking about taking up yoga to help ease their symptoms, but are not ready to commit to spending money on it there are some great free resources on the web relating specifically to yoga for migraines. The ABC-of-Yoga has a great article on migraines with an illustrated list of poses, and directions on how to achieve them, on their website at http://www.abc-of-yoga.com/yoga-and-health/yoga-for-migraine.asp.

Chapter 30: Riboflavin for Migraines

Correcting dietary insufficiencies may help reduce headache frequency for migraine sufferers. Many migraine sufferers find relief by adding vitamin supplements to their daily regimen.

Taking vitamin B2, also known as riboflavin, has been shown in numerous studies to help reduce the number of migraine attacks people suffer from. Initial studies involved a high dosage of 400mg. This is two hundred times the amount of B2 in a typical diet. The high dosage involved caused a rare side effect of vitamin B2 supplementation to show itself, diarrhea.

In 2005, a new study measured the effectiveness of B2 at much lower doses, only 25mg a day. This lower dose was just as effective at reducing migraine frequency as the higher dose used in earlier studies.

Riboflavin has the potential to enhance energy production in brain cells. Migraine sufferers tend to have impaired energy production in cells in their brains and supplementing with riboflavin may help.

Magnesium, another nutrient important to energy production, is also proven to reduce migraine frequency among sufferers. Diuretics, alcohol, and chronic medical conditions all deplete magnesium in the body. Adding magnesium-rich foods to their diet, things like spinach, bananas, nuts, and whole-grain cereals, helps many migraine sufferers restore this vital mineral to their system.

If dietary changes don't help, a dose of up to 400mg of magnesium per day may help. Migraine sufferers should be careful not to overdo it with both dietary changes and supplementation. Signs of magnesium overdosing include drowsiness, lethargy, and diarrhea.

Another potentially helpful supplement is vitamin E. Vitamin E aids in circulation and 400 IU (international units) daily helps many migraine sufferers reduce the frequency of their headaches. Fish oil pills with the right balance of omega-3 fatty acids are believed to lessen the intensity of an existing migraine and help stave them off.

Consult with a doctor before adding any supplements to your regular treatment plan.

Chapter 31: Reflexology for Migraines

Say the word migraine and most migraine sufferers will reflexively cringe in remembered pain, their last headache still vivid in their memory. Say the word reflexology to them and you will likely get a blank stare. A recent (2006) study in Denmark indicates that migraine sufferers who get more familiar with reflexology are less likely to cringe reflexively at the mention of migraines.

What is reflexology?

Reflexology is a massage technique based on the idea that every part of the human body has a corresponding point on the sole of the foot. Reflexologists believe that massage and stimulation of these points on the foot can relieve tension, pain, and stress in the corresponding parts of the body.

In the Danish study involved a mix of migraine sufferers and people experiencing chronic tension headaches. Approximately 90% of the people who participated in the study admitted to taking prescribed medication in the month prior to the study specifically for their headaches. After the study, 19% of participants said they were able to stop taking medication for their headaches thanks to the treatment.

The study involved a course of six to eight treatments with monthly follow-up treatments thereafter for a period of six months. At the conclusion of the six months 23% of the study participants said they were completely cured and no longer having headaches. Fifty-five percent of the participants noted marked improvement in their condition— headaches were less frequent and less severe. A remarkable 78% of the study participants saw an improvement in their condition.

At a follow-up check three months after the conclusion of the study 23% of the migraine sufferers stated they were cured. About 41% said they felt their quality of life was improved.

The treatments were most effective on younger patients and those who had been experiencing migraines for a shorter period of time.

Chapter 32: Butterbur for Migraines

Migraine sufferers would prefer not to have migraines at all. If headache cannot be eliminated, reducing the number of migraine episodes they experience would certainly be an improvement. It would be even better if it could be done without synthetic pharmacologicals.

Migraine sufferers, meet butterbur (Petasites hybridus). Butterbur is a shrub native to southwestern Asia, Europe, and northern Africa. It is not what's above ground that makes it interesting though, it's the root. Several studies have shown that daily doses of extract of butterbur root reduced the frequency of migraine episodes by approximately 50% in almost 80% of the participants.

Butterbur is used in Europe and Asia, but only in the last decade have American doctors looked at it as a viable herbal preventative for migraine sufferers. Double blind, placebo-controlled studies conducted in 2000, 2002, 2003, 2004, and 2005 all confirmed the herb's efficacy.

Migraine frequency reduction ranged from 37% - 62% among study participants, with almost no side effects. The only side effect reported was minor gastrointestinal upset, and that was in a small portion of both the herb and placebo groups. Butterbur is currently considered to be safe, as of this writing, to take with other migraine medications. A healthcare professional should always be included in the decision to add herbal products to any treatment regimen.

Crude butterbur contains pyrrolizidine alkaloids (PAs). These alkaloids are known to be toxic in humans, particularly to the liver. When choosing butterbur, make sure the product is labeled PA-free.

The amount of alkaloids in butterbur root is minimal, less than 0.01% concentration. Most butterbur treatment regimens recommend taking the supplement for a maximum of for to six months. If migraine frequency increases, it is safe to take again for another 4-6 months, but at least a month needs to separate each course of treatment.

Chapter 33: Chiropractic Care for Migraines

Chiropractic care is a safe, non-invasive way to relieve migraine suffering without the use of medication. Chiropractic migraine treatment is not for everyone, but it may be particularly useful for patients who cannot use prescription medication due to other risk factors.

Migraine headaches are idiopathic. This means that despite the last century's advances in medical science their cause is still unknown. A number of theories exist to explain migraines. They include a possible serotonin deficiency in migraine sufferers, genetics malformations, and arterial swelling in the cranium.

A common chiropractic theory is that subluxations in the muscles at the base of the skull and the neck cause, or contribute to, the formation of migraine headaches. Subluxations are tense areas in the muscles adjoining the small bones of the upper spinal column. On an x-ray, the bones appear to be in the correct place and medical doctors often miss the tension in the muscles. A chiropractor gently manipulates the spine to relax these subluxations.

Chiropractors offer two varieties of care for migraine patients, straight chiropractic and mixed chiropractic. Straight chiropractic only involves manipulation of the spine and spinal subluxations. Mixed chiropractic care combines traditional manipulation with other complementary techniques. The focus in mixed chiropractic is to reduce overall neck strain and tension.

Researchers at Northwestern College of Chiropractic in Minnesota recently compared chiropractic care with drug therapies for migraines and chronic tension headaches. The study was published in the Journal of Manipulative and Physiological Therapeutics. Two hundred eighteen headache patients were given either drug therapy or regular chiropractic care. Both groups reported a 40-50% reduction in headache pain at the end of the study.

Follow ups four weeks after discontinuing all care showed only the chiropractic group still enjoying the pain reduction the treatment initiated. Only 20-25% of the drug therapy patients were still benefiting from their treatment at this follow up.

Chapter 34: Cognitive Behavioral Therapy for Migraines

Some migraine sufferers are fortunate enough to experience prodromal symptoms that let them know a migraine is coming. It isn't much, but it allows them to plan for the down time they know they are about to enter into. A migraine sufferer who has learned cognitive behavioral therapy can utilize the same prodromal symptoms to short circuit their migraine headache.

Cognitive behavioral therapy for migraine sufferers is aimed at recognizing at consciously manipulating the role that a patient's behaviors play in the development of their headaches. Together the patient and therapist will determine how the patient behaves when they feel a headache coming, or when the pain starts for those who do not experience prodromal symptoms. They then develop alternative behaviors to try in the same situation in hopes that changing the behavior will change the migraine.

In cognitive behavioral therapy, the doctor or therapist works with the migraine sufferer to:

* Identify the problem behavior to be modified. This is often done by having the patient maintain a headache diary.
* Establish a treatment goal. This is usually not the total elimination of the migraine, but a step along the way, such as learning to relax around potential migraine triggers.
* Create a new behavioral pattern to try to affect change.
* Monitor the patient's reaction to the new behavior and check for environmental factors that may be influencing the behavior.

Common behavioral therapy techniques include:

* Desensitization
* Positive Thinking
* Reframing
* Role-Playing and
* Self-Talk

Cognitive behavioral therapy can be helpful by itself, but is especially helpful to patients who are also on preventive drug therapies. A 1989 study found that clinic-based and minimal-therapist contact behavioral therapy had roughly equal success rates, both initially and upon follow-up six month later. Minimal contact therapy is therefore an effective, affordable treatment alternative for migraine sufferers.

Chapter 35: Applying Heat or Cold for Migraine Relief

Many migraine sufferers relieve the pain of a migraine with the judicious application of heat or cold. This type of pain abatement is particularly popular with people trying to minimize or avoid prescription medication use, especially among pediatric patients and their families.

Below are a few techniques that can help ease the pain of a migraine. Not all techniques work for all patients. While some migraine sufferers find comfort in cold, at least as many are more uncomfortable in the presence of cold. The same is true of heat used for pain relief—for some it helps, for others it makes the pain worse.

Apply a compress, hot or cold, to point on the head where pain is most severe. This is frequently on the temple where a large artery runs, or in front of the ear, another arterial locale.

For patients who feel their migraine pain "stabbing into the back of the eye", a damp cloth (warm or cool) laid over the eyes often provides relief. As a side benefit, covering the eyes in this manner also eases the discomfort of photosensitivity for many patients.

Taking a hot or cold shower with the water directed at the head and neck is another method to try, as is taking a warm (neither hot nor cold) bath. The latter is further enhanced with the use of appropriate aromatherapy techniques.

Some patients find relief in by alternating hot and cold cloths at the point where the migraine pain is most intense. Sometimes hot and cold used simultaneously can ease the pain. A migraine sufferer may apply a cold compress on their forehead while at the same time soaking their feet in a container of warm water.

Rarely are patients simultaneously sensitive to both hot and cold, but it should be watched for.

Chapter 36: Hypnotic Migraine Relief

Hypnosis is not just an entertainer's trick to please and amuse crowds. Hypnotherapists are helping migraine sufferers ease their pain. Sometimes they are even able to relieve other migraine symptoms like vomiting and sensitivity to light and sound.

The hypnotist's goal is to relax patients into a trancelike state in order to access their subconscious mind. A good therapist will then place gentle suggestions in the subconscious that will help migraine sufferers' deal with their pain by changing how they perceive it.

Rather than focusing on pain perception, some hypnotherapists work with patients to learn to identify and avoid their personal migraine triggers. This can be doubly effective for migraine sufferers who smoke if it is one of their triggers. Hypnotherapy has been a recognized smoking cessation technique for decade.

Some patients enjoy this type of therapy so much, since it usually very relaxing, that they decide, either on their own or with the aid of a therapist, to learn self-hypnosis. Oxford Hypnotherapy has a free downloadable book and audio course available on their website for people who would like to learn more about self-hypnosis. You can find it at http://www.hypnos.info/pages/freeselfhypnosis.html.

Hypnotherapy is an excellent option for patients who do not respond to traditional migraine therapies. It is a great alternative for those who are either sensitive to migraine medications or are unable to take them for medical reasons. Hypnotherapy is highly recommended for women trying to avoid medications during a pregnancy or while breastfeeding.

Hypnosis is not magic. Patients are not under a spell or in the thrall of the person who puts them into the trance. Hypnotherapy is an interactive process between therapist and patient.

Hypnotherapy should only be undertaken with a certified hypnotherapist. To find a good one, check with the American Association of Professional Hypnotherapist (online at www.aaph.org) or the National Board for Certified Clinical Hypnotherapists (www.natboard.com).

Chapter 37: Exercise to Ease Migraines

The relationship between exercise and migraines is quixotic. Science says that exercise, by promoting the regular release of endorphins, the body's natural pain controllers, should help ease the frequency and severity of migraines. Many migraine sufferers claim that their attacks are triggered by physical exertion. Who is right?

Like many other aspects of migraines, the answer is contradictory because both groups are correct. Strenuous exercise can cause migraines in people who are prone to them. Regular exercise can reduce the frequency and severity of migraine headaches as well as increasing overall health and wellness.

Regular exercise reduces the risk of developing cardiovascular diseases like high cholesterol and high blood pressure. It also helps improve sleep patterns and relieves stress. All of which can subtly affect the likelihood of migraines.

Migraine sufferers who gave up exercise as a headache trigger should try again. Common exercise migraine triggers are things like:
* Not eating properly before exercising and causing a dramatic drop in blood sugar to occur
* Not taking in enough fluid and becoming dehydrated while exercising
* Starting a new eating plan and a new exercise plan at the same time
* Attempting strenuous exercise without warming up properly

To pinpoint exertion-related migraine triggers, migraine sufferers should keep an exercise log. It should include specific information:
* Time of day when exercising
* Last meal prior to workout
* Fluid intake
* Medication details
* Whether or not a headache occurred during or after the workout

The best type of exercise for migraine sufferers is regular, moderate aerobic exercise, at least 30 minutes three times a week. Recommended activities include:
* Power Walking
* Jogging
* Cycling
* Swimming
* Dancing

Any new exercise plan needs at least six weeks to find out if it has an effect on migraines.

Chapter 38: Migraine Trigger Elimination Dieting

Science can't explain why so many migraine sufferers claim that there is a link between certain foods or beverages and their headaches, but they do. Sadly, the food triggers are different for each migraine sufferer—it's not like someone who needs to lower their cholesterol and the doctor tells them to eat egg whites and lose the bacon, migraine sufferers have to figure out their triggers on their own. The best way to do this is with an elimination diet.

 The first step in any elimination diet is to put together a suspect list. A migraine sufferer has had a headache the day after every football party for years. What is served? Who hosts? What items never change from party to party? If it doesn't happen every time, what was different? Did someone else make the potato salad this week? List the suspects and move to step two.

This is the hardest step in an elimination diet. Until a suspect is identified, everything from the meal that seems to trigger a headache must be eliminated. Then the dieter can add items back into their life, one at a time, until they identify a trigger. Once the trigger is identified, it can be avoided.

Do not stop with the first trigger identified. Most migraine sufferers have multiple triggers. If an elimination diet is going to help someone, he or she needs to identify all the triggers.

For many migraine sufferers, the trigger is not a single food, but a combination of foods. For example, avocados trigger migraine sufferer A and B is okay with them. However, when B eats guacamole he gets a headache every time. Why? Guacamole is made up several common triggers including avocado, citrus juice, seasonings, and vinegar. B may be okay consuming any one of these alone, but combine them and its sure formula for a headache.

Chapter 39: Prophylactic Migraine Medications

Doctors sometimes prescribe a daily medication to reduce the duration and frequency of migraine attacks. These medications are called prophylactic or preventive therapy. There are several classes of drugs approved for use as prophylactic migraine treatments.

Beta Blockers
No one knows how beta blockers prevent migraines, but they seem to. Beta blockers commonly used in migraine therapy include propranolol (Inderal), nadolol (Corgard), metoprolol (Lopressor, Toprol XL), atenolol (Tenormin), and timolol (Blocadren).

Tricyclic Antidepressants
Tricyclic antidepressants (TCAs) prevent migraine headaches by altering two of the neurotransmitters, nor epinephrine and serotonin. Since migraines and depression are considered comorbid conditions they are a particularly good fit for many migraine sufferers. TCAs that have been used in migraine therapy include amitriptyline (Elavil), imipramine (Tofranil), doxepin (Sinequan), and imipramine (Tofranil).

Side effects of TCAs include increased heart rate, blurred vision, difficulty urinating, dry mouth, constipation, and weight change.

Anticonvulsants
Antiseizure medications, also called anticonvulsants, have been used to prevent migraine headaches. Like many prophylactic migraine treatments, it is not known how they work, they simply do. The anticonvulsants gabapentin, valproic acid, topiramate, and phenobarbital have all been used in migraine therapy.

Calcium-Channel Blockers
Calcium-channel blockers (CCBs), in addition to blocking calcium from entering the muscle cells of the heart, appear to block a serotonin uptake. It is the latter that has caused their occasional use in preventing migraines. The CCBs used in preventing migraines are verapamil (Calan, Verelan, Isoptin), diltiazem (Cardizem, Dilacor, Tiazac), and nimodipine.

Antiserotonin Agents
The antiserotonin agents, methysergide and methylergonovine can be used in migraine prophylaxis, but their potential side effects are so severe, including retroperitoneal fibrosis (scarring of tissue around the ureters that carry urine from the kidneys to the bladder) and scarring around the lungs, that they are rarely used in this capacity.

Chapter 40: Poison the Pain – Botox for Migraines

Botox can make you look better. Did you know it could also make you feel better? Moreover, we are not just talking about self-esteem here. Migraine sufferers looking to smooth out some wrinkles in their foreheads discovered a happy side effect of the cosmetic treatment—fewer migraines.

Botox, botulinum toxin type A, is a neurotoxin most famous for its use in smoothing wrinkles. The FDA originally approved it in 1989 as a treatment for eye muscle disorders, and the cosmetic use came later.

Botox is thought to work by weakening or paralyzing the muscles by stopping or slowing the release of the neurotransmitter acetylcholine (ACh). ACh transmit the signal from nerve to nerve to cause muscle contraction. When ACh production is inhibited muscles relax, including those that cause wrinkles.

Acetylcholine is also a neuromodulator. This means it affects how other neurotransmitters function. ACh alternately excites and sedates nerve endings, and it is this ability to suppress excitability that may help migraine patients. One theory on migraine causes is based on the idea of a cascade of nerve excitement in the brain that agitates the arteries in the brain. This in turn stimulates nerve sensitivity, which further inflames the artery, in a vicious circle.

Botulinum toxin is the same agent produced by spoiled food that causes botulism. When used medically, the toxin is injected straight into the muscles and not absorbed into the bloodstream. The dose of toxin required to cause botulism is significantly larger than used in medical applications.

Like most prophylactic migraine treatments, Botox injections may take several weeks to become effective. Depending on the study, Botox has proven effective at reducing migraines for 60-90% of study participants. Injections should be given at least three months apart and the effects should last ten to thirteen weeks. Botox is not currently FDA approved as a migraine treatment.

Chapter 41: Toradol - When Migraine Pain Won't Stop

Doctors give migraine sufferers medications to reduce the frequency or duration of their headaches, and some to stop the pain when they feel a headache coming on. Sometimes, though, the pain is resistant and heavy-duty pain medications are needed.

Non-prescription NSAIDs, non-steroidal anti-inflammatories, help a lot of people relieve their migraine pain, but when they are not enough doctors may offer a prescription version. Toradol (ketorolac) is a prescription-strength NSAID doctors can dispense to migraine sufferers with moderate to severe pain that is resistant to other pain relievers. It is available in a tablet form, but is usually dispensed in emergency rooms and injected for migraines

Toradol has a host of potentially dangerous side effects patients need to be aware of and should be used with caution. It can cause nausea, drowsiness, dizziness, itching, diarrhea, fluid retention, and perforation or bleeding of the gastrointestinal tract.

It should not be taken by migraine sufferers who are allergic to other NSAIDs or aspirin. Patients with a history of gastrointestinal bleeding, high blood pressure, or a history of kidney and liver problems should avoid ketorolac. It should be avoided by pregnant women and the elderly as well.

Patients who have been unsuccessfully trying to treat their migraine at home with over the counter NSAIDs need to let their doctor or emergency room staff know. Ketorolac should not be administered until other NSAIDs have cleared the body to avoid potential overdose-related complications.

Due to potentially dangerous drug interactions, patients need to let their doctors know about all their medications, not just ones taken for migraines. Toradol should not be given to anyone currently taking blood thinners, tranquilizers, diuretics, lithium, and particular types of antidepressants, methotrexate, or ACE inhibitors for blood pressure.

Toradol may offer relief when no relief from the pain can be found, but should be taken with extreme caution.

Chapter 42: Using White Noise To Treat Migraine Symptoms

Phonophobia, an extreme sensitivity to noise is one of the most unpleasant side effects of migraine headaches. Doctors can't help with this sensitivity, but there is hope. The phonophobia most migraine patients experience is particularly sensitive to very loud noises or sudden noises. White noise can help.

What is white noise? If you've seen Pollyanna, you know that white light is actually composed of light from every color of the spectrum. White noise is a combination of all audible frequencies. The sounds are spread evenly across the frequency band so that no one single sound or frequency stands out. When the frequencies are mixed they cancel each other out and create a deadening effect.

This deadening effect has helped some migraine sufferers by masking other, more painful sounds during a headache. One of the best natural ways to relieve migraine pain is to sleep through it. Migraine pain makes it hard to fall asleep, especially when you add in the photosensitive and phonosensitive elements. A white noise machine or recording can help soothe the sensitivity long enough to allow a migraine sufferer to fall asleep.

For migraine sufferers who experience prodrome symptoms, symptoms that let them know a migraine is coming, white noise can help stave off a headache. For many migraine sufferers, noise is a headache trigger and the noise canceling properties can help stop a headache by removing the noise trigger from the environment. One article even suggested that white noise machines be made available to migraine sufferers at work as a prophylactic measure to reduce lost time due to headache.

Some people find relief from migraines by staring at the visual white noise on a television screen set between channels or with the cable unplugged. Some report that the migraine disappears completely. Those who use visual white noise recommend doing so with the sound off.

Chapter 43: Thermal Biofeedback and Migraines

Thermal biofeedback is an effective technique used by many migraine patients to reduce the pain intensity and frequency of their headaches. This is especially true of pediatric migraine sufferers, particularly those who have entered puberty.

Pregnant migraine sufferers can doubly benefit from biofeedback. It enables them to avoid potentially dangerous medication during their pregnancy. Second, a 1996 study showed an 80% reduction in headache frequency and intensity among pregnant migraine sufferers.

Thermal biofeedback, sometimes referred to as psycho-physiological feedback, is a treatment modality used to instruct people in the conscious control of their body temperature. Patients achieve control through a combination of visualization (guided imagery), voluntary relaxation, and mechanical feedback.

A 1983 study tested the effects of three different medication-free techniques, thermal biofeedback, frontalis EMG biofeedback, and relaxation training, on migraine sufferers. Patients using each technique experienced improvement in their migraines, but the thermal feedback patients appeared to experience the greatest success rate and were more able to sustain the effect long term.

Patients are attached to a temperature sensor, usually on the hand, during instruction in thermal biofeedback. This sensor allows them to see the effect of their attempts to consciously control their temperature and change their methodology as needed to achieve the desired result.

Training in thermal biofeedback is usually provided by a psychologist or an alternative medicine provider in an office setting, and then practiced by the individual alone. Patients interested in learning this technique should screen instructors thoroughly since there is currently no licensing requirement for those who provide it.

At-home thermal biofeedback practice is frequently more successful in children because they tend to be more imaginative than adults. To utilize this treatment successfully, patients must be very motivated and diligent in practicing it. Some adults can only achieve thermal control when guided by an instructor and are unable to practice the technique alone.

Chapter 44: Balancing Chakras to Soothe Migraines

The word chakra is Sanskrit for wheel. The chakras are the seven primary distribution points for the energy in the body that run from the base of the spine to the crown of the head. They are also called the psychic centers of consciousness. Migraines may be a side effect of a blocked chakra or unbalanced chakras. Migraines can be eased, and possibly cured, without the aid of the prescription drugs by clearing and balancing the migraine sufferers' chakras.

Each chakra is the energy focal point for a different part of the body or body system and affects the energy flow of both physical energy and emotions. The two chakras most concerned with migraines are, naturally, in the head.

Ajna, Sanskrit for command, is the sixth of the seven primary chakras. It is also known as the brow chakra or the third eye. It is in the center of the forehead between the eyes. This chakra is linked to psychic ability as well as the more mundane pineal and pituitary glands. Migraines are considered, by some, to be a sign of a weak or blocked Ajna chakra. When balanced the Ajna chakra is a deep indigo color.

Sahasrara, or the thousand-petalled lotus, is the seventh of the primary chakras. It is also known as the crown chakra since this chakra is on top of the head and includes the entire crown area. This chakra works with the root to balance energy throughout the body. Stress, fatigue, sleep problems and migraines are all associated with an unbalanced crown chakra. When balanced the Sahasrara is violet.

Meditation, visualization, and color therapy are all excellent ways to balance the chakras of the head. Many people find crystals and semiprecious stones helpful in focusing and balancing their chakras. Check your local library for more information about healing through chakra balance.

Chapter 45: Migraine Abortive Medications

Doctors prescribe two types of migraine medications. One type is designed to help stop a migraine that has already begun. This is called abortive therapy and these drugs work best when taken as soon as the headache begins. The other type is a daily medication designed to reduce the frequency of migraine attacks. This type of medication is called prophylactic or preventive therapy.

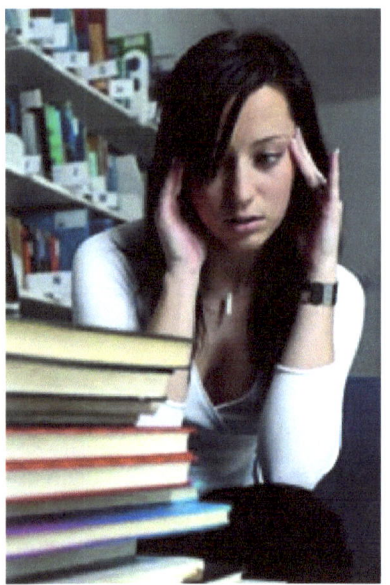

There are two common classes of migraine abortive prescriptions, triptans and ergots.

Triptans (sumatriptan, zolmitriptan, naratriptan, et al.) work by attaching to serotonin receptors on the blood vessels and nerves in the brain. By blocking these receptors, inflammation is reduced and the vessels are able to constrict. This effectively ends the migraine for many. Triptans are available as injections, tablets, and nasal sprays. When used early enough triptans can abort up to 80% of migraine headaches within two hours of taking the medication.

Common triptan side effects are facial flushing, tightness in the chest and/or throat, and skin tingling. Less common, though still not considered serious, are dizziness, drowsiness, and fatigue. The biggest danger of triptans is heart attack or stroke in people with previously undiagnosed heart disease or risk factors like obesity and high blood pressure.

Ergots (ergotamine or dihydroergotamine preparations), like triptans, abort migraines by constricting of blood vessels. Ergots are not as targeted as triptans, however, and cause constriction of vessels throughout the body, not just in the brain. They are not considered to be as safe as triptans and are generally only recommended for patients who are unable to find relief with safer alternatives.

Ergots cause prolonged contraction of the uterus and can cause a pregnant woman to miscarry. Ergots are also much more likely than triptans to cause nausea and vomiting. Ergot brand names include Cafergot, Wigraine, Migranal, and Ergomar.

Chapter 46: Lifestyle Change for Natural Migraine Prevention

Migraine sufferers are turning to non-pharmacological options to reduce the number of headaches they have. Prophylactic drugs aimed at migraine prevention can have many unpleasant side effects and do not work at all for some migraine sufferers.

A migraine sufferers' lifestyle impacts the severity and frequency of the attacks and lifestyle changes, like those mentioned below can prevent migraine recurrence.

Sleep:
Migraine sufferers need to learn how much sleep they need and make sure they do not get too little sleep or too much more than they need. Patients who do not get enough sleep during the workweek who try to make up for it over the weekend may trigger a headache.

Exercise:
Physical exertion in moderation is good for everyone, including migraine sufferers. Establishing a regular exercise routine including at least 20-40 minutes of physical activity a minimum of three times a week, relieves stress that triggers headaches and exercise-induced endorphins are a natural analgesic.

Stress Management:
Migraine sufferers are susceptible to attacks during periods of high stress. If stress is unavoidable, they should build time for stress relief into their routine to prevent a headache. Good stress management techniques for migraine sufferers are massage, exercise, adequate sleep and a healthy diet.

Eating:
Migraine sufferers should eat regular meals at roughly the same time daily and not skip a meal unless it is an emergency. A good, healthy breakfast goes a long way in preventing headaches.

The most important thing is to be consistent with any lifestyle change. Migraine sufferers need regular behavior patterns and they must be applied on weekends and holidays, not just during the week. Getting out of sync two days a week by sleeping in, skipping meals, or staying up late defeats the purpose of lifestyle changes and upsets the balance created by having a pattern the rest of the week.

Chapter 47: Fewer Migraines with Feverfew

Migraine sufferers are looking for headache relief that doesn't come from a drug lab. All too often pharmaceutical migraine solutions have unpleasant side effects, including, ironically enough, headache.

Some migraine sufferers have found help from feverfew (Tanacetum parthenium), a common flower that grows all over Europe and North America. Feverfew plants resemble daisies. They have flat yellow centers with slender white petals on lightly furred stems and small yellow-green leaves. Medical texts going as far back as Ancient Rome list dried and crushed feverfew leaves as a palliative for headaches.

Feverfew is best used in a preventive program. Several clinical trials, all in the past decade, have shown that feverfew, taken two to three times a day, can reduce the frequency of migraine episodes by up to 50% for some people. Several study participants who experienced chronic daily headaches (CDH) plus migraine episodes reported that their daily headaches stopped completely after four weeks of feverfew treatment.

Feverfew, while helpful to some, has a significant amount of potential side effects. Few people experience them, but they can be serious. Any patient wanting to add feverfew to their migraine prevention regimen should consult with their doctor and a licensed herbalist.

Feverfew is available in many forms. It can be homegrown and the migraine sufferer can chew two to three leaves from the plant each day. It is also available in tea, tablet, capsule, and tincture forms. Feverfew in any form can cause mouth ulcers, but they are most common among those that chew the leaves or drink the tea. If mouth sores develop, discontinue use immediately.

Pregnant or nursing women should not take feverfew. Do not give feverfew to pediatric migraine sufferers without consulting a doctor. Feverfew can trigger an allergic reaction in patients with common pollen allergies and should be used with caution.

Chapter 48: Genetic Research into Migraines

Migraine headaches are a huge health problem. In a 2004 report, the World Health Organization (WHO) called migraines and headache disorders a global public health calamity. Migraines and other chronic headache conditions are disabling. In the same report, the WHO ranked migraine as one of the top twenty conditions in the world to cause years of healthy life lost due to disability. Migraines and all other headache disorders combined rank in the top ten causes of disability. As a result of the increasing global recognition of migraine as a health threat, genetic research into the condition has multiplied exponentially in the last ten to fifteen years.

Doctors have long known that a child with two migraine sufferer parent will likely have migraines. A 2000 Danish study using primarily twins indicated that migraines without aura (common migraine) is approximately sixty-one percent genetic, making migraines a partially genetic disease. Family history studies and the Danish study both suggest that migraines are a multi-genomic condition, meaning that several genes or combinations of genes are required for the condition to be inherited.

In a study published in June 2003, Dutch doctors revealed that a particular sub-type of migraine, familial hemiplegic migraine, follows a conventional Mendelian inheritance pattern (simple inheritance) in seventy-five percent of all cases. The same study indicated that common migraine is considerably more complex. Several potential genetic loci have been looked at.

The Genomics Research Centre at Griffith University, Queensland, Australia, reports progress in locating genetic loci for migraines. Researchers have been studying multi-generational migraine sufferers within the same family for years. According to their website, the researchers have identified three different genetic regions on the chromosomes 1, 19, and X that harbor genes which increase migraine susceptibility. This type of research may eventually lead to a genetic treatment for migraines.

Chapter 49: Finding a Migraine Doctor

You have severe, debilitating headaches that cause you to vomit and huddle in a dark room for hours waiting for them to go away. Chances are they are migraines. The only way to know for sure, and start on the path to managing your condition if they are migraines, is to be properly diagnosed.

The first step should always be your regular doctor. One out of every eight people suffers from migraines, so chances are good that your doctor has seen someone who has migraines before. If your regular doctor does not feel qualified to properly diagnose the source of your headaches or discounts your pain, it may be time for a specialist.

Ask your doctor for a referral to a headache specialist. If they do not know anyone, check with your insurance company to see if they have any specialists listed. If that doesn't work (or even if it does), contact your local medical board. You can also try one of the major headache organizations for professionals, not patients, and ask for the name of three or four specialists in your area.

Check with friends and family. The odds are good you know someone with migraines and they may just have a doctor they love. Another good place to ask for a referral is at a local teaching hospital or university.

When you have a few names, call and find out more about the doctor. Some good screening questions to ask the doctor are:

* How long have you been specializing in headache treatment and how often do you treat headache patients?
* Are you certified in your specialty (for doctors in the U.S. and Canada)?
* Do you belong to any headache-oriented professional organizations?
* Do you participate in any kind of continuing education program to stay apprised of the latest research on headache diagnosis and treatment?

Chapter 50: Online Resources for Migraines

Many migraine sufferers feel very alone in their misunderstood suffering, but they are not alone. There are a number of support groups where migraine sufferers can find understanding, information resources, and encouragement.

The American Council for Headache Education (ACHE)
You can find ACHE online at www.achenet.org. Their mission is to educate patients and health care providers about headaches, including migraines. Their website has a wealth of information about migraine diagnosis and research as well as an "Ask the Expert" section staffed by physician volunteers, all of whom are headache specialists.

The World Headache Alliance (WHA)
The WHA's home on the web is at www.w-h-a.org. The WHA is a truly international organization, bringing together the efforts of 38 headache organizations in 26 different countries. This is one of the best sites on the web for current research information and innovative news about migraines and other headache conditions.

Migraine Awareness Group: A National Understanding for migraine sufferers (MAGNUM)
Find MAGNUM on the Internet at www.migraines.org. This site has a lot of good information and is an excellent resource for people wanting to get involved in migraine activism.

The Migraine Trust
The Migraine Trust is an excellent, United Kingdom-based resource that can be found online at www.migrainetrust.org. They are particularly devoted to workplace migraine awareness and activism and put out a newsletter packed with good information.

The Migraine Action Association (MAA)
The MAA's website at www.migraine.org.uk gives visitors a look at the history of one of the oldest migraine support and advocacy groups in the world, established in 1958. The site also has a very inclusive list of local chapters and support groups throughout the UK.

Headaches and Migraines at About.com
A wealth of information and links to lots of other good resources are at http://headaches.about.com.

Conclusion:

Migraine headaches affect millions of individuals around the world. They are extremely painful and hard to bear. Migraines can last anywhere from one hour to three or four days. Within that time, it may literally be impossible for migraine suffers to function properly. Although relief might not come right away, there are many options available that soothe or cure migraine headaches.

A migraine is classified as a serve headache that can often impair one's judgment. When a migraine occurs, suffers regularly experience the following symptoms:

• Sever Headache
• One-sided and frontal headache
• Throbbing headache
• Dizziness
• Nausea and vomiting
• Weakness
• Light and sound sensitivity
• Difficulty seeing and eye pain

Migraine can be triggered by many factors but all of these do not yet have scientific explanations. It includes allergic reactions, perfume odors, stress, irregular sleep patterns, meal skipping, alcohol, caffeine, pills intake, headaches due to tension, foods with tyramine, chocolate, peanut butter, banana, dairy products, and many more.

There are also drugs that can trigger migraine. These include nitrates, theophylline, reserpine, nifedipine, indomethicin, and cimetidine. So watch out for these if you know that you have the tendency to have migraine.

If you are unable to control the pain associated with your migraine headaches, it is extremely important that you contact your physician. Beta blockers, along with other medications, offer quick relief from migraine headaches, however, they are only available with a prescription. If you experience migraines, do not suffer any longer than you need to. Contact your physician or healthcare professional for effective ways to receive relief from your migraine headaches.